This book is dedicated to our hungry, nutritionally deficient children, including those from affluent families. It is our deepest prayer that the knowledge in this book reach every home in every village, town, and city on Earth.

The Magic of Kefir

The miracle food that restores
your inner ecosystem and your health!

From the Body Ecology Healthy Living Series
by Donna Gates
with Linda Schatz

B.E.D. Publications, Inc. Atlanta, Georgia 30305

The Magic of Kefir is written as an information resource and education guide for both professionals and nonprofessionals. It should not be used as a substitute for your physician's advice. Be sure to work with a physician who knows the importance of diet in healing and who has experience in treating Candida Related Complex and other immune disorders. While we endorse *The Magic of Kefir* and related recommendations, you should make your decision based on all the information at hand, knowing that you are the primary force in directing your own life and health.

THE MAGIC OF KEFIR

ISBN: 0-9638458-0-2

Printed in the United States of America

B.E.D. Publications Co.
P.O. Box 550556
Atlanta, GA 30355

Table of Contents

DONNA GATES is a nutritional consultant and an expert on candidiasis and related immune disorders. She has conducted extensive research on how these debilitating conditions affect the body, mind, and spirit. She developed the Body Ecology Diet and tested it on many different people who have all improved their health by following the basic principles of the Diet. She has studied with the top macrobiotic teachers and graduated from Lima Osawa's cooking academy in Japan. She holds an M.Ed. in Counseling from Loyola University and a B.S. in Early Childhood Development from the University of Georgia.

LINDA SCHATZ is a professional writer and editor. She is co-author of *Managing By Influence* (Prentice Hall) and has been a newswriter for ABC News and *Good Morning America*. She also coaches authors on how to write books and book proposals. Her specialties are self-help books in areas such as health, nutrition, and business. Linda holds an M.A. in Communication from Stanford University and a B.S. in Journalism from the University of California, Berkeley.

I am constantly searching for ways to help people recover from immune disorders and to help healthy people stay well and live a longer, happier life. My goal is to have more people enjoy perfect physical, emotional, and spiritual health. My relentless...perhaps even compulsive...search for answers has led me to an exciting and important new yet ancient food. I became interested in this food because it is cultured, it is enzyme-rich, it is a "live" food and, most importantly, it helps to establish and maintain a thriving inner ecosystem.

When I first encountered Kefir years ago, I didn't understand its value. An excellent colon therapist mentioned to me that Kefir, especially goat milk Kefir, has a very beneficial, toning effect on the colon. After a bit of searching, I found a goat farmer and master yogurt and cheese maker, Bob Spotts of Boyertown, PA, who made delicious Kefir. I ordered some and tried it, but was highly skeptical since it was made from milk. Milk sent up a red flag for me. Milk is mucous-forming, feeds yeast, and in Chinese medicine, produces a sticky, "damp" quality. Besides, I had always been lactose intolerant and allergic to milk. So, even though I enjoyed it, I quickly dismissed Kefir as an unimportant food.

Then, as always happens for me, I began to see signs that I needed to open my mind to new possibilities. For example, I happened to turn on television (I rarely watch) and saw a program about fish in a Canadian lake producing mucus to protect themselves as the lake's pH level rose due to acid rain. Several weeks later, I lunched with a friend whose daughter had brought home a book describing how a fish had totally covered itself with mucus when it washed up on the beach, protecting itself until the rising tide returned the fish safely back to sea. I realized mucus can be a protection. After a little more reflection, I remembered that all things in this universe have a positive and a negative side and I had been focusing only on the negative.

I tucked this information away in my mind and, as I began collecting more information about Kefir, more parts of the puzzle fell into place. For example, I knew that, at birth, a newborn has no inner ecosystem and must establish it during the first few months of life, ideally from breast milk. In fact, Nature decrees that mother's milk be available for all offspring of mammals. This milk lays down a bed of clean mucus, allowing friendly bacteria to establish themselves. Breast milk is an excellent source of protective agents such as lauric acid, a powerful antimicrobial that deactivates pathogenic bacteria, yeast, fungi, and some viruses. This protects the baby until the inner ecosystem is well established with positive bacteria and his immune system matures.

Now, as we all know, Nature does not make mistakes. So, as I began to add up all the facts, I realized that: 1) there is both good, clean-quality mucus and toxic mucus, 2) good mucus coats and protects the interior lining of the digestive tract, and 3) unlike yeast, who burrow into the intestinal walls with their tentacles, good bacteria do not have tentacles. They must be caught by this clean mucus where they nestle into their warm,

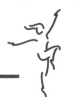

acidic environment, fed by the sugar (lactose) in mother's milk. Mucus, I finally had to admit, was an essential part of a healthy inner ecosystem.

People with candidiasis have a very unhealthy inner ecosystem. They have an overgrowth of fungus or yeast, and very toxic bowels. In order to heal, they must first cleanse the colon and control the yeast overgrowth. Then they must reestablish an inner ecosystem teeming with beneficial bacteria. At this second stage, a victim of candidiasis could be compared to a newborn babe...both must have this vibrant, living inner world if they are going to assimilate nutrients, create a strong immune system, and live a long, fruitful life.

It was becoming clearer to me that Kefir had tremendous healing power. With its laxative effect it helps clean the colon. Its beneficial bacteria and yeast help control the pathogenic yeast and repopulate the colon with a favorable, new life force. And Kefir, being cultured, is much healthier than milk.

It is said that in ancient times Kefir was given to the people of the Caucasus regions as a gift from the gods. Perhaps these gods were watching over mankind and offering us this miracle food at a time we desperately needed it. Now, if only I could learn to make Kefir and test out my theory. The problem was that no one had grains or a starter culture, there was almost no information available, and the few people who knew about Kefir did not want to share their "secrets." Then a miracle happened!

After publication of the first edition of *The Body Ecology Diet*,

I felt drawn to take a spiritual sabbatical to recharge myself and give thanks for the success of the book. I traveled to a sacred area of Japan and attended a ceremony honoring the creation of humanity. A friend from Sendai, Japan, joined me the evening before the ceremony and brought with him Mrs. Kwai, a woman I had never met before. He told me that his friend had felt very strongly compelled to come and bring with her something she thought I needed. Amazingly, it was a little brown pot of Kefir grains cultivating in milk. Mrs. Kwai opened the container and, having brought a strainer, spoon, and another jar, began to show me how to make Kefir.

My prayers were being answered. In amazement I brought the Kefir back to my room, still not fully appreciating what I had been given. I ate the Kefir, loving the taste and feeling a surge of strength after my tiring journey. When I returned home, everything started coming together.

Since Bob Spotts still sold his excellent goat milk Kefir, I began referring many of my students to him. When they began eating it in the morning on an empty stomach with the addition of flax seed oil or Essential Balance Plus™, (and perhaps with stevia, lecithin, and other flavorings) they gradually became much stronger. Now I had something valuable to share, but my next concern was how to make this wonderful Kefir available to more people. Bob Spotts lacked the production capacity to supply Kefir to millions of Americans. And I especially wanted it available for our children, pregnant and nursing women, the elderly, and the millions of us who have had antibi-

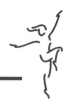

otics, steroids, and cortisone. So I turned my next prayer into a question and a request. "If Kefir is the solution, who will manufacture it for us? Please help!"

My prayer was answered in the form of John Donovan, a handsome, energetic New Zealander whom I met at a Natural Products Expo in California. John's company, The GoodLife Company and Friends, makes a wonderful little "Kefir Kit," a pocket-size device containing Kefir grains to start your own culture. Here's his story:

In the late 1950s, when John was a boy, his mother, Phyllis, was given some Kefir grains. A health enthusiast, Phyllis came to appreciate the benefits of eating fresh, homemade Kefir every day. It became a staple food for her growing family of five children. She now has nine grandchildren and eight great grandchildren, and everyone in the family thrives on Kefir. Phyllis has kept those grains active all these years and believes that her own longevity and that of her husband is largely due to Kefir. John's parents are in their 80s; both are fit, active, lean, and healthy.

John himself was fascinated by the Kefir grains and the alchemy they weave with milks. The commitment he and his wife Julia have to making the world a healthier place led them to establish a company to grow and distribute Kefir grains. John invented a convenient pocket-size Kefir maker which enables anyone to produce fresh Kefir at home. The "GoodLife Kefir Kit" simply floats Kefir grains on milks. It is totally reusable and, properly cared for, never needs replacing.

Now John and Julia travel the world, teaching people about the many benefits of fresh Kefir. By encouraging people to make their own Kefir at home, the Donovans are advocating self-reliance rather than dependence on store-bought goods. The GoodLife Kefir Kit represents their strong commitment to promoting preventive health practices while also preserving our environment. Eliminating the need to buy packaged yogurts and cultured milk at the store eliminates the need for untold tons of plastic packaging and disposal of that packaging.

But the greatest benefit goes to those who eat fresh Kefir every day. This ancient, simple food, made at home so easily and inexpensively, provides a crucial step in the urgent process of reestablishing our health and well-being.

I can't recommend Kefir highly enough. It is a nutritious, incredibly delicious food. If your body is ready for it and you find you tolerate it well, Kefir can be essential to your achieving maximum health and immunity. As you read the information in this book and begin to eat Kefir, you'll realize, too, that it is an ancient remedy for today's modern maladies: a true gift from heaven. Enjoy!

Overview of the Body Ecology Diet

The Body Ecology Diet is a synthesis of seven principles of eating and healing. Those principles form the pillars of the holistic health field. Some of them are thousands of years old, such as the Chinese concept of yin and yang (contraction/expansion). Others, such as the theory of blood types, are more recent.

The Diet weaves these complementary principles together like pieces in a puzzle. They offer a frame-work for healthy eating for the rest of your life. The Body Ecology Diet shows you how to integrate these simple principles into your daily routine. When they are properly implemented, you will see your symptoms disappear and your overall health improve.

The Diet is about restoring your inner health, strengthening your immune system, and establishing a pattern of living and eating well that will extend your vitality for years to come. It provides basic tools to help you achieve a new balance in your life. Anyone, ill or not, can benefit from The Body Ecology Diet.

The Body Ecology Diet shows you how to restore and maintain the "inner ecology" your body requires to function properly. Kefir now plays a starring role in The Body Ecology Diet.

Outer Ecology, Inner Ecology

In the early '70s, Rachel Carson, author of *The Silent Spring*, launched the environmental movement by warning us that we are slowly destroying the ecological balance of our planet by adding chemicals to our crops, particularly DDT. She cautioned us about the pesticides that leach into our food and water supplies, affecting our health and the health of future generations, endangering even the birds that sing in the spring.

In a remarkably similar manner, we are destroying the delicate balance of the ecosystem within our own bodies. This intricate internal ecosystem is inhabited by microorganisms that play a crucial role in keeping us looking young and feeling healthy and strong. These friendly creatures, such as lactic bacteria, reside in the digestive tract. They help strengthen the immune system and assist the body in defending itself against "unfriendly" bacteria and the pathogens that cause disease.

Both friendly and unfriendly microorganisms are always present in our bodies. But when we are healthy, the friendly ones greatly outnumber the unfriendly, keeping our inner ecosystem in balance. However, many factors weaken our immunity and upset this balance: the chemicals we add to our food and to our environment, fast food diets, the stress in our daily lives, and the widespread use of medicines, particularly antibiotics and hormones. When the body is in this weakened state, unfriendly bacteria can multiply quickly, creating symptoms such as headaches, flu, skin rashes, food allergies, and other, potentially more serious disorders.

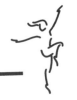

One of the most common types of unfriendly organisms is Candida albicans, a yeast, or fungus, normally present on inner and outer body surfaces. It also co-exists in our digestive tract and in a woman's vagina alongside friendly microorganisms. Yeast must consume sugars to survive. It is an opportunistic organism that rapidly takes advantage of any weakness in our system. So if we're eating improperly, or taking, say, antibiotics, or changing our body chemistry with birth control pills, we are providing the candida with a perfect environment in which to take control. The vagina and the intestines are especially susceptible. For example, only two days on antibiotics can cause candida overgrowth in a susceptible person. When yeast multiplies, it excretes toxic waste products which circulate in the body, further weakening both the immune and the endocrine systems.

The overgrowth of candida constitutes a condition we call candidiasis or Candida Related Complex (CRC). CRC has been linked to many symptoms, including food allergies, digestive disorders, PMS, skin rashes, chronic constipation, recurring headaches, chronic vaginitis, chemical and environmental sensitivities, poor memory, mental fuzziness, and loss of sex drive. CRC occurs side by side with other diseases such as chronic fatigue, cancer, AIDS, Epstein-Barr virus, bronchitis, pneumonia, Multiple Sclerosis, Attention Deficit Hyperactivity Disorder, and immune system deficiencies. Experts estimate that more than 80 million Americans have candidiasis, but the majority don't attribute their symptoms to this modern epidemic.

To reverse this overgrowth of candida, we must restore an inner environment that prevents candida from taking over. This requires two major actions: killing off the yeast and other opportunistic parasitic organisms, and recolonizing the friendly bacteria and beneficial yeast. Both are essential to reestablishing your inner ecology; it won't do any good to reestablish new colonies of friendly bacteria without improving the environment so they can prosper. The miracle food you will read about in this book will help establish that environment.

Most of us begin life with a clean bill of health, a perfect body inside and out. Experts disagree on exactly where a baby's friendly bacteria comes from, but we do know that mother's milk promotes its growth. As breast feeding continues, the bacteria establish themselves in the baby's digestive tract and in the vagina of the female infant. It takes about three months for an inner ecosystem to settle in and, after this period of time, the infant's amount of lactic (friendly) bacteria closely resembles that of the mother.

As the child's inner ecology develops, the beneficial bacteria thrive on natural sugars from breast milk, and then from food, particularly complex carbohydrates. These sugars transform into lactic acid, which the friendly bacteria need to survive. Once the friendly bacteria establish colonies in the intestines, they have created an ideal, self-sustaining habitat, which ideally should endure through adulthood, though for most people it does not. When this habitat changes, we are at risk for disease.

We used to believe that conscientious application of the Body Ecology Diet and all its principles would eventually provide a complete reversal of candidiasis. It's true: many, many users have reported such improvement that they call themselves "cured." They are symptom-free. But others, though they feel much better, tell us that their symptoms return when they stop following the Diet. And for a significant number of people, digestive problems persist or there is unwanted weight loss. This means that the inner ecosystem still is not fully reestablished and needs some additional help. It also means even the healthiest foods may be passing through the body without their nutrients being adequately absorbed.

The digestive tracts of people with candidiasis are deficient; they do not assimilate food properly. The undigested food ferments, causing bloating and gas. When you are not digesting properly, you may also be gaunt-looking, underweight, and have constant food cravings. When you begin following the proper food combining rules and start cleansing with the Diet, you naturally lose weight as the toxins and the bloating leave your body. Some people are thrilled with the weight loss. But for those who started out on the thin side, it can be a concern. The solution is to restore the integrity of the digestive tract as quickly as possible so it can begin to assimilate food properly, allowing the body to attain its optimal weight. Remember, you are not well until your inner ecosystem is in balance. That is why we wrote this book.

Without detracting from the importance of The Body Ecology Diet, probiotics, raw cultured vegetables, and **VITALITY** *SuperGreen™*, our superfood formula, there is another wonderful food that will help you enter the final phase of getting well, restore the integrity of your digestive tract, and add to the effectiveness of everything else you've done so far. That food is Kefir.

Kefir is a cultured and microbial-rich food that helps restore the inner ecology. It contains strains of beneficial yeast and beneficial bacteria (in a symbiotic relationship) that give Kefir antibiotic properties. A natural antibiotic—and it is made from milk! The finished product is not unlike that of a drinking-style yogurt, but Kefir has a more tart, refreshing taste.

The Body Ecology Diet recommends avoiding dairy products because they contain a milk sugar called lactose that feeds yeast and creates mucus. But Kefir does not feed yeast, and it usually doesn't even bother people who are lactose intolerant. That's because the friendly bacteria and the beneficial yeast growing in the Kefir consume most of the lactose and provide very efficient enzymes (lactase) for consuming whatever lactose is still left after the culturing process. Yes, Kefir is mucous-forming, but only slightly so if you follow some simple food combining rules (more on the food combining principles later).

And here's the capper: the slightly mucous-forming quality is exactly what makes Kefir work for us. The mucus has a "clean" quality to it that coats the lining of the digestive tract, creating a sort of nest where beneficial bacteria can settle and colonize. This makes the other probiotics you may be taking even more potent: They now have a better chance to take hold and proliferate in your intestines, helping you really "get your money's worth." By the way, Kefir can be made from any type of milk, including milk made from soy, coconut, or rice. More on this later.

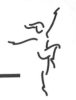

You're probably wondering, "What does Kefir look like?" Kefir is made from gelatinous white or yellow particles called "grains." The grains contain the bacteria/yeast mixture clumped together with casein (milk proteins) and polysaccharides (complex sugars). They look like pieces of coral or small clumps of cauliflower and range from the size of a grain of wheat to that of a hazelnut. Some grains have been known to grow in large flat sheets that can be big enough to cover your hand. No other milk culture forms grains...making Kefir truly unique.

Once the grains ferment the milk by incorporating their friendly organisms into the final product, you must remove these grains with a strainer before drinking the Kefir. The grains are then added to a new batch of milk, and the process continues indefinitely.

You may have seen television ads for yogurt that portray very old people from Bulgaria or some area near Russia attributing their long lives to their daily consumption of yogurt. Kefir is similar but more therapeutic (see below). It is also well-known and loved in Poland, Hungary, Finland, Norway, Sweden, Denmark, and Switzerland. Muslims believe that the prophet Mohammed granted them Kefir grains, the essential base used in fermenting the milk, cautioning that it would lose its strength if given to other people. So the preparation of Kefir remained a secret for a long time. The term Kefir may come from the Turkish word "keif," meaning "good feeling," or the sense of well-being you experience after eating it.

Marco Polo mentioned Kefir in his account of his Eastern travels. But after that, for nearly five centuries, Kefir was forgotten in the West. Interest in it revived in the early 19th century, when tuberculosis sanitariums used it as part of their treatment. It is still given for TB therapy in Europe and Russia; a typical patient consumes one and a half to two quarts a day. Chinese medicine teaches us that the lungs and large intestine are paired, so if Kefir benefits the large intestine, it follows that it would also benefit the lungs.

Donna has always had weak lungs and had frequent lung infections as a child and as a teenager. She had three major lung "cleansings" after starting to eat Kefir, and after each one, she noticed an improvement in her lungs...especially in her ability to breathe more deeply. Quite surprised and thrilled at this unexpected improvement in her health, she can now exercise with much more endurance than before and has plenty of energy to get through her busy days.

They look alike. Both are fermented foods, creamy, and white. But there the similarities end and dramatic differences begin. Kefir is more "drinkable," more tart and more effervescent than yogurt. Yogurt and Kefir contain completely different types of beneficial organisms. Yogurt generally contains transient beneficial bacteria that do not stay and colonize in the intestinal tract, but do help to keep the area clean, and do provide food for the beneficial bacteria that remain as permanent residents.

Kefir contains several major strains of friendly bacteria (such as Lactobacillus Caucasus, Leuconostoc species, Acetobacter species, and Streptococcus species), and it also has strains of beneficial yeast, (such as Saccharomyces kefir and Torula kefir). The yeast account for less than 10 percent of the total, but this is an important ratio for those of us looking for protection against pathogenic yeast. These good yeast dominate, control, and even destroy the bad ones.

Pathogenic yeast actually live below the first few layers of mucosal lining in the intestinal tract, so they are very difficult to reach. Kefir does a great job of reaching them. And the several strains of friendly bacteria in Kefir prevent pathogenic bacteria from trying to set up housekeeping in our intestines. So if you are exposed to pathogens such as E. coli, you have a better chance of fighting them off.

Kefir, experts believe, has more therapeutic value than yogurt. Its very active yeast and bacteria provide more nutritive value than yogurt since they excel in digesting the foods you eat and in keeping the environment of the colon clean and healthy.

Yogurt is made by adding a starter culture to milk and gently heating it to a certain temperature. To make Kefir, you must start with the "grains" and no heating is required. This means that if you can obtain a reliable source of fresh, raw milk, you can retain enzymes that would normally be destroyed by the heat of pasteurization. Kefir "cultures" at room temperature for about 24 hours, right on your kitchen counter.

Kefir grains cannot be manufactured; they occur naturally. So you must obtain your grains or "starter" from an ancient, original strain. Kefir grains are eternal. With proper care, Kefir grains can be used over and over and last a lifetime.

After your inner ecology is restored, you may find that you digest yogurt well and want to make use of its friendly bacteria. But choose Kefir first. The friendly bacteria and yeast in Kefir are crucial to the restoration process. We think of them as a SWAT team moving in quickly to begin the therapeutic process, efficiently doing the job they were created to do.

You may see a product in the store that claims to be Kefir, but read the label carefully. Unless it has strains of friendly bacteria *and good yeast*, it is not true Kefir. As far as we know, Lifeway Foods, Inc. of Skokie, IL, is the only commercial company that makes and sells true Kefir. That's why Donna has worked so hard to find a reliable, inexpensive source of real Kefir grains so you can make it yourself...fresh and delicious.

Why Kefir Aids Digestion

According to Beatrice Trum Hunter's *Fact Book on Yogurt, Kefir and Other Milk Cultures* (now out of print), Kefir has a very low curd tension. This means that the curd breaks up very easily into extremely small particles. (Yogurt curds either hold together or break into lumps.) The small particle size of the Kefir curd facilitates its digestion by presenting a large surface on which the digestive agents can work. This ease of digestion means that Kefir can be particularly helpful for infants, convalescents, the elderly, or people with weak digestive systems.

Kefir stimulates the flow of saliva, increases the flow of digestive juices in the gastrointestinal tract, and stimulates peristalsis (the wave-like movements of your digestive tract). Because of this, it is recommended as a post-operative food, since many abdominal operations cause the temporary cessation of peristalsis, accompanied by gas pains. Kefir also has a laxative effect and is used extensively in Russia and its neighbors to relieve chronic constipation.

Benefits as Friendly Bacteria

With more than 400 different species of beneficial bacteria living inside a healthy gut, why not give them the optimal environment? As we've said, Kefir lays down a foundation of clean mucus so these beneficial bacteria have a place to thrive. When you add probiotics like Body Ecology's EcoRenew (friendly organisms purchased from your health food store), they too will find a receptive home much more quickly when a favorable environment has already been created.

The fact that you can easily make Kefir fresh every day or so in your own kitchen means that its friendly yeast and bacteria are readily available to do their job in your intestinal tract.

After you restore the balance to your inner ecology using the Body Ecology Diet, cultured vegetables, probiotics, and Kefir, your intestinal tract will be teeming with friendly organisms. Then you will be better able to enjoy some foods containing natural sugars (fruits, whole cereal grains, the sweeter vegetables such as yams and parsnips), and you may tolerate that occasional binge on really sugary food such as a piece of cake or candy. The beneficial bacteria gobble up the sugar for themselves first, leaving little to carry into the rest of your body. Of course, we are not endorsing foods with refined sugar, but it certainly doesn't hurt to have yourself prepared and "well-armed."

If you are a parent worried about all the sugary foods your child wants (and usually gets), Kefir is especially useful for

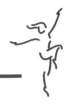

establishing and maintaining a strong immune system in your child. To make a Kefir treat that kids love, add the natural, sweet-tasting herb stevia, some non-alcoholic fruit flavorings or vanilla, and/or Omega Nutrition's new, butterscotch-flavored Essential Balance Junior™ oil. We will explain later why this unrefined oil is so good for you.

Kefir keeps the small and large intestines clean and free of parasites. Once in the large intestine, the beneficial bacteria create lactic acid that balances the pH level there. In this acidic environment parasites and other unfriendly organisms cannot survive. Kefir's beneficial yeast and bacteria are ready to ambush any parasite eggs or larvae before they have a chance to establish themselves and multiply.

With its .02% alcohol content (produced by the yeast), Kefir is acidic when you make it; yet it becomes alkaline-forming in the body once you eat it. This means that the overall quality of the blood remains slightly more alkaline and we remain healthy. When our blood becomes too acidic, we become ill. In **The Body Ecology Diet** (see Chapter 6, "The Principle of Acid and Alkaline"), we explain the healing value of alkaline-forming foods.

The friendly bacteria and yeast in Kefir provide a good advance team for other probiotic cultures like acidophilus and bifidus. Kefir "clears the land" and establishes clean, healthy sites for new colonies of friendly bacteria. When the new settlers arrive (the friendly bacteria you buy in your health food store or generate internally by eating cultured vegetables), they remain and thrive, ensuring you a far better return on your investment.

New research has found that stomach ulcers are often caused by a pathogenic bacteria called *Helicobacter pylori.* Expensive antibiotic therapy is now being used to kill this bacteria. Kefir, with its natural antibiotic properties, may prevent such ulcers. Remember, pharmaceutical antibiotics kill *all* bacteria, both the good and the bad, so it is important to remain on the Body Ecology Diet if you must take antibiotics, using it and Kefir to rebuild your inner ecosystem.

Benefits Regarding Nutrition

Kefir contains *complete* protein with all the essential amino acids. By the time you drink Kefir, its friendly bacteria have already partially digested the protein, making it much easier for you to digest. High amounts of protein are critical to healing, and your body must have adequate minerals in order to assimilate the protein. Kefir provides these, too. Abundant calcium and magnesium are found in Kefir.

Tryptophan, an essential amino acid found in Kefir, combines with the calcium and magnesium to help calm the nervous system. Some people call Kefir "Nature's tranquilizer" or "Nature's Prozac." Its calming effect is great for people who are high-strung or nervous, for hyperactive children, or for people with sleep disorders, such as the elderly. The body

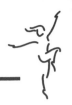

converts tryptophan into serotonin, an important chemical called a neurotransmitter; increased serotonin levels induce sleep and prohibit waking during the night. This conversion is helped along by Vitamin B6, which is also abundant in Kefir.

Kefir has ample phosphorus, the second most abundant mineral in our bodies. Phosphorus is important in utilizing carbohydrates, fats, and proteins for growth, cell mainte- nance, and energy. A phosphorous deficiency can result in the loss of appetite.

Kefir and the B Vitamins

There are 22 known B vitamins; so, as you can imagine, they facilitate many functions in our bodies. Many people take B vitamins for stress reduction, but these vitamins are also vital to other areas of health. We'll discuss a few of them here.

People with candidiasis are usually deficient in the B vitamins and in Vitamin K because the body's use of these vitamins depends on adequate levels of friendly bacteria in the intestinal tract. When Kefir is included in the diet, your body should soon be able to manufacture sufficient amounts of these need- ed bacteria. Vitamin K promotes blood clotting, encourages the flow of urine, relieves menstrual cramps, increases vitality and longevity, and enhances liver functioning.

Kefir provides biotin, another B vitamin, which is missing in people with candidiasis. Biotin is a coenzyme that assists in the manufacture of fatty acids and in the oxidation of fatty acids and carbohydrates. Without biotin, the body's production of essential fatty acids is impaired. Biotin also aids in the body's assimilation of protein and other B-vitamins: folic acid, pantothenic acid, and B12. A deficiency of biotin can cause muscular pain, poor appetite, dry skin, lack of energy, or depression and a distressed nervous system.

Kefir is an excellent source of Vitamin B12, which is essential for longevity. It is the only vitamin that contains essential mineral elements. It cannot be made synthetically but must be grown, like penicillin, in bacteria or molds. B12 is necessary for the normal metabolism of nerve tissue and for red blood cell formation. B12 builds immunity and has been used to increase energy and counteract allergens. It is also required for normal growth and is important for fertility and during pregnancy. Plus it works along with folic acid, another member of the B-complex, in facilitating the synthesis of choline. [Choline is a fat and cholesterol dissolver and plays an important role in the transmission of nerve impulses. It helps regulate kidney, liver, and gallbladder functions and aids in the prevention of gallstones.]

B12 helps the placement of Vitamin A into body tissues by aiding carotene absorption or Vitamin A conversion. It also aids in the production of DNA and RNA, the body's genetic material. B12 needs to be combined with calcium during absorption to benefit the body properly; of course, Nature has provided for that in Kefir.

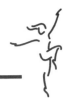

B12 is found in substantial amounts only in animal protein, so doctors often warn vegetarians to supplement their diets with B12. However, Paul Pitchford, in *Healing with Whole Foods*, maintains that anyone with weak digestion, whether vegetarian or meat-eater, can become deficient in vitamin B12. Other factors also deplete the body of B12: birth control pills, antibiotics, stress, liver disease, and chronic illnesses.

Kefir is rich in thiamin (Vitamin B1), also known as the "morale vitamin" because of its beneficial effects on the nervous system and on mental attitude. Thiamin is linked with enhanced learning capacity, growth in children, and improvement in the muscle tone of the stomach, intestines, and heart. It is essential for stabilizing the appetite and improving digestion, particularly of carbohydrates, sugar, and alcohol.

Benefits Regarding Your Overall Health

Kefir helps stop food cravings because the body feels nourished as an inner balance is achieved and nutritional deficiencies are corrected.

Kefir provides a "sour" taste. Chinese medicine teaches us there are five tastes necessary for balance in the body; the sour taste is not commonly found in our American diet.

The skin prospers from Kefir. It will become moist and creamy and, over time, you will notice a refinement of the pores. You can use Kefir externally to help moisturize your skin; yet, it is beneficial for oily skin too. Fermented milks contain lactic acid which is one of the naturally occurring Alpha hydroxy acid (AHA) so popular in the cosmetic world today. You'll love experimenting with our skincare recipes in the last chapter.

Kefir is cooling to the body, so it is ideal to eat when you have a fever or any other condition of body heat.

After taking antibiotics (which we hope that you and your loved ones can avoid), Kefir is very useful for reestablishing friendly bacteria in the intestines. Kefir is "Nature's antibiotic." Using it helps reduce the need for antibiotics in the future.

Kefir's friendly bacteria automatically show up in the vagina, or you can implant them more directly as a douche.

While colonic therapy helps cleanse pathogenic yeast from the large intestine, such yeast colonize in the small intestine as well. Fermented foods like Kefir and raw cultured vegetables have a cleansing effect on both intestines. Once these are free of pathogens, the liver is able to function much better, releasing its toxins into a clean colon as it was designed to do.

Kefir helps produce a more pleasant breath, healthier bowel movements, and sweeter-smelling stools. And it can eliminate flatulence!

The Kefir grains we recommend come from The GoodLife Company and Friends in New Zealand. When they first started manufacturing Kefir, they produced far more than they needed at the time. So they sold the excess to local pig farmers. Soon these pigs began commanding top prices on the market—the meat was tender, lean, and tasty. The inner ecosystems of the pigs had benefited from the Kefir, making them healthier and the farmers wealthier.

Give Kefir to your pets (mammals only) regardless of their age. Kittens, cats, puppies, dogs, pigs, and rabbits thrive on it. Older pets with health problems (skin conditions, body odor, eye problems, and constipation) respond well to one bowl of Kefir each morning. Kefir helps detoxify the body, improving the health of the liver and preventing more serious conditions of toxicity like cancer.

Donna's dog, Curly, loves goat milk Kefir. When she first got him, he had been in a kennel for two years and had not been well cared for. He had a very "doggie" odor, and his urine was thick and very dark yellow. After four days on the Kefir, he had a clean, fresh smell. The Vitamin K in Kefir promotes the flow of urine. That first week he began to urinate more frequently, and his urine became very healthy, too.

Some people thrive on Kefir right from the start and others may need to proceed more slowly. Remember that people with candidiasis often lack milk-digesting bacteria, so you may have to build up your "tolerance" of Kefir. Start with about four ounces in the morning on an empty stomach. Every second day increase the amount until you are able to drink a full eight ounce glass.

If you are just beginning the therapeutic version of the Body Ecology Diet's health recovery program, it might be best to wait three to six months before introducing Kefir. You may first need to clear your body of accumulated toxins and see your symptoms disappear. Moreover, people with candidiasis have what Chinese medicine calls the condition of dampness. Dairy products can lead to even more dampness and excess mucus. There are several ways to counter this tendency:

1. Wait three to six months until your condition of dampness has dried up a bit.

2. Eat Body Ecology Diet foods, which are drying.

3. Drink a lot of water; it helps pass the mucus through your body more quickly.

4. Be sure to get adequate exercise, since the heat of physical activity helps burns up mucoid accumulations.

5. Use proper food combining techniques to make Kefir less mucous-forming.

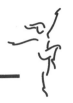

6. Make Kefir from raw milk if possible; the enzymes help break down the fats and proteins and are less mucous-forming.

7. If available, make your Kefir from goat milk rather than cow milk. It forms less mucus, is more digestible, and is usually free of antibiotics or other drugs now common in cow milk. Goat milk has more calcium, magnesium, phosphorus, and potassium than cow milk. (It contains no folic acid, however, so pregnant and nursing mothers should consider a folic acid supplement.) Some people think goat milk has a strong, or unpleasant taste. This occurs only when the goats are victims of poor hygiene, the milk is no longer fresh, the goats have a tainted food supply or a mineral deficiency, or if a male goat has been allowed near a female goat. If you would like to learn more about the benefits of goat milk, see *GOAT MILK MAGIC* by Dr. Bernard Jensen.

As a dairy product, Kefir should be eaten alone, on an empty stomach, or combined with:

1. raw or lightly steamed vegetables (Try a salad with our Kefir dressing recipe, or use our recipe to make a Kefir dip for raw veggies.);

2. acid (sour) fruits such as strawberries, lemons, limes, grapefruits, pineapples, cranberries, or blueberries.

Kefir smoothies are especially delicious and very popular as a morning breakfast for our children. In the beginning the non-alcoholic flavorings taste great, but as your child becomes well, you can add acid fruits. Simply blend Kefir, your favorite berries or flavorings and stevia. A little unrefined flax seed oil, Essential Balance Plus™, or Essential Balance Jr.™ (all made by Omega Nutrition) is a "must" for children...especially those with eczema and Attention Deficit Hyperactivity Disorder.

To insure that Kefir is not overly mucous-forming, do not combine it initially with proteins or starches.

Around the world, however, Kefir is eaten throughout the day, even as a digestive aid after a meal. Once your inner ecosystem is restored (anywhere from three months to a year), you may experiment and want to try Kefir at the end of a meal, even though it is more mucous-forming at this time. See what works for you. Some people think that eating Kefir about an hour before bedtime helps them relax and fall asleep.

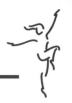

In *The Body Ecology Diet* chapter on food combining, we recommend you wait three hours after eating dairy foods before dining on protein or starches. However, because Kefir's protein is pre-digested and the friendly yeast and bacteria speed up digestion, you need only wait about 45 minutes to an hour before eating something else.

So have Kefir as your first food of the day and follow the directions in the next chapter for additions to this morning "cocktail."

Contents of a Spectacular Kefir Drink

Make your Kefir with the freshest milk possible, then add as many of the following ingredients as you wish:

- Up to 1 tsp. of unrefined flax seed oil or Essential Balance Plus™ oil. These oils give us the essential fatty acids most of us lack and that our bodies are not able to manufacture. EFAs are a major constituent of the body's cell membranes. They help maintain the integrity of these membranes, thus preventing invasion by viruses, bacteria, yeast, and other parasites. They are also vital to the brain, more than half of which consists of EFAs.
NOTE: We now have available Essential Balance Junior™, (made by Omega Nutrition), a butterscotch flavored oil that is especially appealing to kids.

- Lecithin to taste. Lecithin assists in the digestion of fat. If you make Kefir from skim milk, the only fat will come from the unrefined oil. However, the beneficial microorganisms prefer a little fat, so 2% or whole milk makes a better Kefir.

- Fiber, such as Nutri-Flax™.

- Probiotics, if you are taking them currently.

- Natural flavorings or herbs, such as stevia, nutmeg, cinnamon, or non-alcoholic vanilla or fruit flavorings (peach, strawberry, lemon, lime, raspberry, orange, tangerine).

Prescription for Healing

Many popular diet books (*The Zone, Protein-Power, The Atkins Diet,* and *The Carbohydrate Addict's Diet*) recommend a ratio of 40% carbohydrates (e.g., fruits and vegetables), 30% protein, and 30% fat. If you have been following these recommendations, you'll be delighted to know that you can make a meal with this ratio in a Kefir shake, using the above ingredients. People who are healing need a lot of protein, but not necessarily from animal foods, which can be difficult to digest and put a strain on the liver and the colon. The protein in dairy foods such as Kefir and in micro-algae such as that in our **VITALITY** *SuperGreen*™ is much more accessible and useful to the body. Studies have found that combining Kefir and organic, unrefined oils that contain omega-3 and omega-6 essential fatty acids (flax seed oil and Essential Balance Plus™) creates a special lipoprotein that has amazing healing properties. It activates prostaglandins that are critical catalysts for proper hormone function. This benefits our energy, metabolism, skin color, the functioning of the lungs, liver, and heart, and greatly enhances longevity.

Our brain prospers from good nutrition, too. It especially needs the essential fatty acids found in the good oils we recommend and from amino acids, the building blocks of protein found in Kefir.

Some people believe that milk and dairy products should be eaten only by newborns, and that, since no adult animals in the wild drink milk, we adult humans shouldn't either. Others have an ethical objection to dairy products. You need to decide for yourself.

Perhaps you will achieve such great results with Kefir that you will want to continue it indefinitely. Or you may want to use it for a short period of time, being mindful of its mucous-forming effects. Or maybe two to three times a week is best for you. Studies show that cultured foods such as our raw cultured vegetables, Kefir, or miso and tempeh in the more traditional Oriental diet, are key components in a genuinely healthy diet. It is wise to keep colonizing the intestinal tract with beneficial bacteria. Research shows that beneficial bacteria disappear from the stool once probiotic therapy is discontinued.

We would not recommend anything that we haven't found to be superior in helping people heal, but we also know how important it is to trust the wisdom of what your own body tells you. Learn to listen to its signs and signals.

Kefir for People with Special Needs

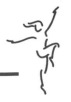

Because Kefir offers such an excellent source of nourishment, it can be particularly useful for these groups:

- Pregnant and nursing women.

- The elderly, who typically have a low level of beneficial bacteria in their intestines, low levels of calcium, and higher than average sleep disorders.

- Children with ADHD (Attention Deficit Hyperactivity Disorder). As "Nature's tranquilizer," Kefir has a calming effect on these kids. A recent study found that ADHD children are deficient in essential fatty acids, so a combination of Kefir and unrefined flax seed oil or Essential Balance Junior™ would be terrific for them.

- People with AIDS or herpes. Yeast overgrowth frequently accompanies both these conditions. The lack of a healthy inner ecosystem also means that food is not digested well; mild to severe nutritional deficiencies are common. Easy-to-digest and nutrient-rich Kefir drinks blended with organic, unrefined and fresh-pressed essential fatty acid (EFA) oils can be an extremely valuable food. Research has shown EFA deficiencies are common in people with viral infections. Adding these Omega-3, Omega 6, and GLA oils to the protein-rich Kefir really helps. In Chinese medicine, viral infections are considered to be a "heat" condition. Kefir has a cooling effect and works well here, too.

Constipation

Even though Kefir traditionally is recommended as a laxative, a small percentage of people find it constipating. This may be because they lack the enzymes to digest the milk protein (casein) in the Kefir. Fortunately, an enzyme extracted from the pineapple stem (bromelain) is very effective at digesting casein. So, if you have this problem, simply take bromelain purchased from your health food store until your inner ecosystem is restored with enough protein digesting bacteria to handle the casein. Do not use enzymes with hydrochloride acid or protease, since they destroy the beneficial bacteria.

If you become constipated after adding Kefir to your diet, ask yourself these questions:

- Am I eating enough fiber? Kefir lacks fiber, so be sure to eat plenty of high fiber foods: vegetables, salads, raw cultured vegetables, and the Body Ecology grains.

- Am I following the food combining rules?

- Am I eating too much Kefir and skipping other meals? Since Kefir is so delicious and is the perfect "fast food" it is easy to overeat it, skipping essential high fiber meals.

- Am I eating sugary foods and flour products? Both are constipating.

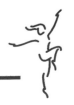

Older, more acidic Kefir also is more "binding". We have found this more acidic Kefir to be beneficial in cases of diarrhea, which is common in AIDS or in cancer patients undergoing chemotherapy or radiation.

Teeth

A final reminder: brush you teeth after you eat Kefir. Its bacteria produce an acid condition in the plaque that can lead to decay without proper care (just as any food left in the mouth without proper rinsing and care can lead to decay).

Vitamin C

If you have a cold or other condition that creates a lot of mucus, such as an ear infection, put an immediate but temporary stop to your Kefir consumption and start taking therapeutic doses of Vitamin C (several thousand milligrams per day, to bowel tolerance). Kefir is so powerful as a digestive aid that when it is present in the intestines, it may prevent Vitamin C from reaching the bloodstream through its stimulation of peristalsis. The Vitamin C is thus in danger of passing through the body before it can have its beneficial effect.

The Convenient Way

At Body Ecology Diet, we are now making available the unique "Goodlife Kefir Making Kit" from Australia. It is a clever little device that contains starter grains encased in a small cone. The cone has a "floater top" that functions like a buoy, allowing the Kefir Maker to float on top of your milk while it cultures. You save time by eliminating a whole step of straining the grains. The GoodLife Kefir Maker is small, inexpensive, and comes with easy, complete directions. Ask your local health food store to order it for you or:

Call toll free

1-888-KEFIR 4U

The Traditional Way

You can make traditional Kefir yourself by following these slightly more complicated instructions:

What You Will Need:

    Medium to large bowl
    Fine mesh strainer
    1 quart glass jar or GoodLife Kefir Pot™
    1 quart or liter of milk (raw, pasteurized, low-fat or whole)
    2-4 Tbsp. fresh Kefir grains or purchase a Yogourmet™
        starter pack and use 1/2 pack - *available at health food stores*

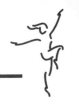

1. Put Yogourmet™ starter culture of Kefir grains into the glass jar of The Goodlife Kefir Pot ™, adding a small amount of room temperature milk. Mix until dissolved.

2. Pour in the remaining milk and cover.

3. Place on counter top and let sit at room temperature for 18 - 24 hours. When a toothpick can stand up straight in the mixture, it is ready for the next step.

4. Pour the Kefir through the strainer and stir with a metal spoon. The liquid will drain through into the bowl, leaving the grains in the strainer. Refrigerate the liquid until ready to eat. This liquid is the Kefir.

5. As the liquid Kefir is stirred through the strainer, you will see grains appearing in the strainer. Rinse them off in the strainer under running (preferably filtered) water. Add these grains to a new quart (or liter) of fresh milk. Repeat steps 3 and 4.

A Special Note

Grains will not appear in your first several batches of Kefir. It will take three or more times before you will see any tiny, cauliflower-shaped grains left in the strainer. So until they appear, simply add 1/4 cup of liquid Kefir from your current batch to the new batch.   This 1/4 cup of Kefir will be your "starter" for future batches. Watch carefully when you strain your Kefir for the tiny new grains to appear. Begin to add them back into each new batch and watch them grow larger and multiply. Soon you won't need that 1/4 cup of "starter" ever again. Your grains will continue to grow and multiply to the point where you will have more than you need and will want to share them with a friend.

Kefir has been called the champagne of milk. Different milks create different tastes. The first requirement is that your milk source be as fresh as you can buy. Organic milk that is free of antibiotics and hormones is also desirable. Clean, raw milk would be best, because it contains enzymes that help you digest the valuable protein, fats, and minerals in the milk. But in America, only a few states still allow the sale of raw milk. This is because our mass production and distribution methods cannot ensure the milk's safety unless it is first pasteurized to destroy pathogenic bacteria. Unfortunately, the high-heat pasteurization process also destroys those valuable enzymes. One of the wonderful benefits of Kefir, however, is that its friendly yeast and bacteria are such powerful producers of enzymes that they help compensate for the lack of pasteurization. You can culture Kefir literally from any kind of milk: Cow (2%, whole, buttermilk, sour cream), Goat (very fresh goat milk makes terrific Kefir), Sheep, Soy, Coconut, Rice.

Do not use lactose-reduced milk, because lactose is the milk sugar that the friendly yeast and bacteria consume as their food. The microorganisms also fancy a little fat, so Kefir made from 2% or whole milk (not skim milk) is better.

As you experiment, you will determine which are your favorite flavors. If you end up with a sour-tasting or distasteful batch from time to time, simply discard it, rinse the cone and grains, and start over. You haven't failed. Maybe the milk was not fresh enough, or it came from a farm you are not familiar with, or maybe you just don't like that flavor.

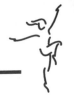

Facts About Raw Milk

Raw milk is no longer available in most of the United States; however, several states still sell raw milk. Today, milk frequently contains pathogenic bacteria and is pasteurized or heated to a high temperature where these bacteria are destroyed. Unfortunately, the enzymes that help digest the valuable protein, fats, and minerals in the milk are also destroyed.

If milk is taken from animals, using clean equipment, and if the animals are well cared for, pathogenic bacteria are not a serious problem. Today, however, in our world where mass production is more important than our welfare, animals are kept in stressful conditions, fed poor-quality foods, and given hormones and antibiotics. Obviously, they cannot produce the high-quality milk of decades ago.

We have found that the freshest milk possible makes the most delicious Kefir. Raw milk obtained from a reliable, sanitary source is absolutely the healthiest. If you cannot obtain raw milk, don't despair. Look for organic, pasteurized, but very fresh cow or goat milk that has no BHT, antibiotics, or other hormones. You probably can only find this quality of milk in your health food store. Check the dates on the milk container, and speak with the store employees. Make certain that the milk comes from a local organic dairy that makes frequent deliveries.

One of the wonderful benefits of culturing milk is that even if you must use pasteurized milk, the good yeast and beneficial bacteria in the Kefir are such powerful enzyme factories that they help compensate for the pasteurization.

With a tablespoon of mature grains, it takes about 24 hours to turn 8 -10 ounces of milk into Kefir at a room temperature of 64º - 86º F. (18º - 30º C). More milk requires a longer setting time or more grains. In winter or if your room is cool and drafty, we suggest placing the culturing milk in a cupboard or cabinet.

Kefir grains multiply quickly and too many grains can cause the milk to culture more quickly than you may want. When you have more grains than you need, separate some out and share with a friend.

If you make more Kefir than you or your family can consume in a day, it stores well in the refrigerator for several weeks. It will, however, become more acidic as it ages and you may not like the taste. If this happens simply add fresh milk to your refrigerated Kefir and let it sit out on the counter for several hours. This brings down the acidity.

Traveling with Your Kefir

Why not take this delicious and nutritious food with you when you travel! The GoodLife Kefir Making Kit™ makes this easy. Carry the kit in a small jar with enough milk so it floats. When you get to your destination, start a new batch of Kefir with fresh milk.

You can also buy organic milk packaged in aseptic cartons so it doesn't need to be refrigerated. Not only is this a blessing for travelers, but other groups could also benefit, such as campers and back-country hikers. People who prepare survival kits in case of disasters like earthquakes or floods could include Kefir tablets and aseptic packaged milk. Kefir would be a treasure in such emergencies.

Juniper Valley Farms of Jamaica, NY makes shelf stable organic milk in aseptic packages that lasts for months without refrigeration. It is ideal for traveling or emergency food supplies. Their phone number is (718) 291-3333. Your health food store can order the 1 quart cartons from: Stow Mill (East Coast), Tree of Life (Northeast and Southeast), Mountain People, Nature's Warehouse (West Coast).

Remember, Kefir combines well with acidic fruits and raw, lightly-steamed, non-starchy vegetables. In addition, to the recipes you will find here, you might try variations on the Kefir drink we've already mentioned. Or consider Dr. Bernard Jensen's favorite: Kefir, carrot juice, and almond butter blended into a delicious shake. For kids, try pouring Kefir mixed with a fruit flavoring, lecithin, and Essential Balance Jr.™ oil into popsicle molds and freezing it to make an appealing snack.

Basic Kefir Dip

Ingredients:

1 cup Kefir
1 clove garlic, minced
1 tsp. Body Ecology's Essential Balance Plus™ oil
1 tsp. apple cider vinegar
Herbamare™ to taste

1. Mix all ingredients well.

2. Season to taste.

3. Chill and serve.

Variations: Grated cucumbers, carrots, zucchini, watercress, parsley, or cultured vegetables can be added. Healthiest if served with raw or lightly-steamed, non-starchy vegetables.

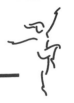

Cool Kefir Dressing (No Oil)

Ingredients:

2 cups fresh Kefir
1 heaping Tbsp. fresh parsley, chopped
1 heaping Tbsp. fresh chives, finely minced
1 heaping Tbsp. fresh lemon zest, finely chopped
1 heaping Tbsp. fresh garlic, finely chopped
1 tsp. sea salt
1/4 tsp. Herbamare™
1/2 tsp. xanthan gum

1. Combine all the ingredients (except xanthan gum) and blend thoroughly.

2. Slowly add the xanthan gum and continue to blend until mixture has thickened.

3. Full flavor will develop after 6 - 8 hours.

Note: Combine with non-starchy vegetables in raw salads. Dairy products combine best with non-starchy vegetables and acid fruits. Don't hesitate to add a little flax oil or Essential Balance Plus ™ (made by Omega Nutrition) to this recipe. The latter is especially delicious and adds a balance of omega-3, omega-6, and GLA essential fatty acids.

Homemade Kefir Cheese
a.k.a. Pot Cheese or Quark

Ingredients:

1 liter plain Kefir
pepper
garlic, minced
thyme, finely chopped
oregano, finely chopped
basil, finely chopped
chives, finely chopped

1. Place a square, double piece of cheesecloth in a large colander, and turn the Kefir in it. Bring up the four corners of the cheesecloth, and tie them together with string. Tie the bag to a ruler or long wooden spoon, and suspend over a large bowl. Allow to drain for 24 hours at room temperature.

2. Untie the bag, and place in the refrigerator to chill.

3. Mix in the garlic and herbs to taste.

4. Sprinkle in snipped chives prior to serving.

Note: Makes 1 to 1-1/4 cups of very creamy low-fat cheese.

Kefir Skincare Recipes

Kefir is wonderful for all skin types. Adding flax seed oil or Essential Balance Plus™ greatly enhances these recipes.

Gentle Exfoliator

A gentle exfoliator for the face and body

Ingredients:

3 tablespoons almond meal (ground almonds)
1/3 cup Kefir

Mix the ingredients together well and apply to the face and body. Leave on for quarter of an hour. Add water and scrub off gently, rinsing with warm water. This is especially good for sensitive skin.

Elderflower & Kefir Lotion

A great all-purpose moisturizer

Ingredients:

4 tablespoons Kefir
2 tablespoons of Elderflower infusion
1 tablespoon apricot oil
2 tablespoons almond oil
1 drop of geranium oil

Make the elderflower infusion as follows: add 1 teaspoon of dried herbs to one cup of boiling water. Strain to remove the herb after five minutes and then allow the infusion to cool. Mix in all other ingredients well by placing in a glass jar with a lid and shaking. Use day or night as a moisturizer for normal to dry skin.

Kefir & Peach Mask

A great mask for most skin types

Ingredients:

1 large ripe peach, skinned
1 teaspoon honey
1/8 cup Kefir
1/2 teaspoon of fine clay

Cut the peach into chunks. Blend it for a brief time and then add the honey. Add enough Kefir to make into a creamy, spreadable consistency. If you do not have a blender, this can be mixed by hand. Leave this mix to sit for two hours, then push it through a sieve and add the clay to make into a paste. Apply to the face and neck, avoiding the eye area. Leave on for twenty minutes and then wash off with warm water.

Properties of Skincare Ingredients

Kefir is rich in alpha hydroxy acids. It softens the skin. Good for balancing both dry and oily skin.

Almond Meal has good emollient properties, and acts as a thickener for cleansing masks. It nourishes and heals the skin.

Peach regenerates tissues and restores the acid balance to the skin.

Honey is high in vitamins and potassium. It is well-known for its healing properties. It moisturizes and softens the skin.

Elder Flower contains an oil which is astringent and gently stimulates the skin. Used to fade freckles and whiten the skin.

Apricot Oil is rich in vitamin E and good for replacing lost oils in the skin and hair.

Geranium Oil is soothing and good for reducing swelling.

Almond Oil is especially good for very dry skin.

- For maximum health, take Kefir on an empty stomach.

- To obtain a microbial-rich, potent Kefir, make a new batch every day or two. Use the freshest milk you can find to ensure high-quality and good flavor.

- Kefir is the healthy equivalent of a "fast food." It provides a filling meal that is nutrient-rich and easy to digest. Its high liquid content makes it an ideal breakfast food.

- Kefir will help you "get your money's worth" out of the probiotics you are using. Making Kefir is inexpensive, and it should be used as one of the first steps in restoring your inner ecology. It will help establish a foundation of beneficial bacteria; then you can add the more expensive probiotics from your health food store.

- Thanks to the availability of The GoodLife Kefir Kit, Kefir is now easy to make at home.

- You can make Kefir from any kind of milk: cow, goat, mare, or sheep, or even soy milk. For a different taste, try making it from buttermilk or sour cream.

- If you are allergic to lactose, don't worry. The yeast and bacteria in Kefir digest the milk sugar lactose. Any remaining is taken care of by the lactase enzymes. After reestablishing your inner ecosystem, you may find that you can more easily digest other dairy foods.

- Kefir is delicious and healing—what more could you want?

Body Ecology Products & Publications

Our Organic, Unrefined Oils

Essential Balance Plus™

Essential Balance Plus Jr.™

Flax Seed Oil

Olive Oil

Pumpkin Seed Oil

Safflower Oil

Handmade Coconut Oil

Other Body Ecology Products

Vitality SuperGreen™

White Stevia Powder

EcoRenew Chewable Probiotic™

GoodLife Kefir Kit™

Handmade GoodLife Kefir Pot

Apple Cider Vinegar

Publications

The Body Ecology Diet

by Donna Gates with Linda Schatz

The Magic of Kefir

by Donna Gates with Linda Schatz

Body Ecology

P.O. BOX 550556 • ATLANTA, GA 30355

CALL 1-888-KEFIR 4U or 1-800-4 STEVIA